GW00889826

Baby Sleep Training

A Healthy Sleep Schedule For Your Baby's First Year

- What to Expect New Mom -

Lisa Marshall

LISA MARSHALL

Copyright © 2021 Lisa Marshall & Giovanni Antonelli

All rights reserved.

This eBook is provided with the sole purpose of providing relevant information on a specific topic for which every reasonable effort has been made to ensure that it is both accurate and reasonable. Nevertheless, by purchasing this eBook, you consent to the fact that the author, as well as the publisher, are in no way experts on the topics contained herein, regardless of any claims as such that may be made within. As such, any suggestions or recommendations that are made within are done so purely for entertainment value. It is recommended that you always consult a professional prior to undertaking any of the advice or techniques discussed within.

This is a legally binding declaration that is considered both valid and fair by both the Committee of Publishers Association and the American Bar Association and should be considered as legally binding within the United States.

The reproduction, transmission, and duplication of any of the content found herein, including any specific or extended information will be done as an illegal act regardless of the end form the information ultimately takes. This includes copied versions of the work, both physical, digital, and audio unless express consent of the Publisher is provided beforehand. Any additional rights reserved.

Furthermore, the information that can be found within the pages described forthwith shall be considered both accurate and truthful when it comes to the recounting of facts. As such, any use, correct or incorrect, of the provided information will render the Publisher free of responsibility as to the actions taken outside of their direct purview. Regardless, there are zero scenarios where the original author or the Publisher can be deemed liable in any fashion for any damages or hardships that may result from any of the information discussed herein.

Additionally, the information in the following pages is intended only for informational purposes and should thus be thought of as universal. As befitting its nature, it is presented without assurance regarding its prolonged validity or interim quality. Trademarks that are mentioned are done without written consent and can in no way be considered an endorsement from the trademark holder.

Publisher: Giovanni Antonelli
Author: Lisa Marshall
ISBN: 979-8725542653

DEDICATION

I would love to dedicate this book to my family, my friends and
to you, my source of inspiration…

CONTENTS

YOUR FREE GIFT

Thank you for purchasing this book. Click on this link to download this free tool.

http://bit.ly/BabySelfSooth

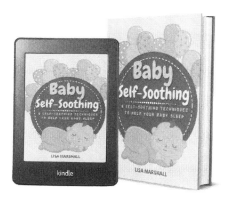

This tool is a useful resource to help your baby being able to self-soothe themselves to sleep. We've compiled some tips to help make the process as quick as possible!

Note: If you have purchased the paperback format then you need to type this link into your browser search bar.

"People who say they sleep like a baby usually don't have one."
—*Leo J. Burk*

INTRODUCTION

First off, congratulations on your new bundle of joy! Or, if you're reading this book in preparation for the birth of your new baby, congratulations on the imminent arrival of your little treasure!

Having kids is a remarkable paradox when you think about it. On the one hand, it's one of the most common roles on the planet. At the same time, it's one of the most personal, unique, and life-changing experiences in the world because no two children are alike, and no set of parents is the same.

However, there's one common denominator that holds for all parents. Parenting, especially for the first time, is one of the hardest jobs you will ever do - and you can't quit halfway through!

So, Mommy and Daddy, let me prepare you for your parenting journey with this summary of what to expect: Caring for a newborn is a sanity-challenging labor of love. It's one of the most fulfilling experiences you will ever know but oftentimes, it can also be the most frustrating. Don't panic; I'm not trying to scare you. Caring for your baby during the first year of his or her life can be relatively painless with some foreknowledge and preparation.

Why This Book?

There are hundreds of parenting books out there and most of them are probably pretty good. However, most baby books try to cover everything and can leave you overwhelmed with too many details. This one is different because it's going to focus on one specific aspect of a newborn's life: sleep.

The biggest challenge you will face in the first six months of your child's life is sleep - namely, your baby's fitful sleep patterns and your sleep deprivation. Newborns have to be fed every couple of hours round the clock, as well as changed, bathed, cuddled, kissed, and a million other things. For new parents especially, it's a total upheaval to your previously well-ordered, quiet life, and normal sleep suddenly becomes an elusive dream.

This is why you can easily spot a new mom or dad. Red eyes, dazed expression, and haggard features are sure signs that the new baby has kept Mom and Dad up all night.

Hundreds of funny anecdotes are related to sleep-deprived moms and dads during those first months. There's the spaced-out dad who drove to work on Saturday before realizing it was the weekend, or the mom who turned on the washer and dryer but forgot to put the clothes in. There are stories of groggy parents putting dirty diapers in the oven or pouring breast milk into their morning coffee. You will no doubt have your own funny stories to tell, but hopefully not too many, because the underlying effects of sleep deprivation can be quite serious. This book will help you avoid these issues.

Sleep deprivation can take its toll on your mental and physical health. More than ever, you need every ounce of energy to look after your newborn as well as focusing on your job, home, and other family responsibilities. Getting enough sleep is vital to maintaining balance and being able to enjoy the amazing first months of your baby's life.

So, how are you going to do this? The simple answer is, by instilling great sleep habits into your baby very early on.

This book is not going to rely on empty platitudes or complex theories and methods. It will provide you with simple, concrete steps and tips on how to train your newborn to sleep soundly so that you can get a good night's rest.

Among other things, this book will cover:

▓ Understanding a baby's sleep patterns during the first months of his life.

▓ How to set the perfect sleep routine.

▓ Powerful settling techniques to help your baby fall asleep.

- Night weaning and phasing out night feeds.

- Sleep routines when you're traveling.

- The ideal sleep environment for your baby.

- Sleep safety tips.

- Detecting sleep problems.

Most parents think that fatigue and lack of sleep go hand in hand with a new baby, but this powerful guide will prove otherwise. Quality sleep for Mom, Dad and baby is possible and will make all the difference in your parenting journey.

From the moment your baby arrives into the world to the moment he takes his first steps, speaks his first words, and begins to bloom into an independent-minded toddler, it's a rollercoaster ride all the way. Exhilarating, thrilling, and sometimes scary. But don't worry, you are going to be amazing parents, and it all starts with a good night's rest...

CHAPTER 1

UNDERSTANDING SLEEP

Think of your brain and body as if it were a hotel room. When you leave the room for the day, housekeeping bustles in and sets the room to rights. They vacuum, change the sheets, replenish toiletries, and put a nice little mint on your pillow. You come back to a fresh, clean room. A similar process of "housekeeping" takes place when we sleep. This is why good sleep is vital for both you and your baby.

Naturally, we all have a general understanding of what sleep is. What we often forget is that sleep is a complex process that's vital to our overall health. Your first step to instilling good sleep habits in your child is to have a deeper understanding of the underlying functions of sleep. This chapter will give you a basic overview.

The Function of Sleep

Just 50 years ago, science believed that sleep was a passive process, meaning that the brain became dormant during sleep and that many of our body functions slowed down. Today, science has discovered that as sleep sets in, our brains and bodies begin an amazing process of healing and regeneration.

Here are some of the things that happen while we sleep:

- During sleep, the brain works to maintain and create neural pathways that help us make memories, learn, and retain learning.

- Sleep allows the immune system to regenerate and replenish white blood cells and other substances necessary for fighting infection and disease (you may have noticed that when you go for a few days without sleeping well, you often come down with a cold). In other words, good sleep promotes a healthy immune system.

- During sleep, your body flushes out toxins that have accumulated throughout the day. It also attacks and destroys germs.

- Sleep helps regenerate neurons, the nerve cells that communicate with each other to regulate various brain and body functions.

- Sleep balances the mood and helps with stress management.

- Heart rate and blood pressure decrease during sleep, allowing the heart to rest.

- Sleep allows your body to regulate and balance blood sugar levels.

- Sleep promotes the regeneration and repair of cells and tissues throughout the body.

The Stages of Sleep

There are five stages of sleep through which an adult transitions during a typical night. These stages are the following:

Stage 1: This is when you start to feel drowsy and begin to transition into sleep. This stage normally takes between 5-10 minutes, and your heart rate starts to slow down.

Stage 2: The scientific term for this stage is non-REM (rapid eye movement) sleep, which means light sleep. You sleep restfully with relaxed muscles but may be easily awakened by external sounds. You may also move your body frequently. This stage lasts for several hours of the night.

Stage 3: This is the deep rest stage where you sleep heavily and your body does not move at all.

Stage 4: This is the very deep sleep stage where you enjoy the most relaxing and restful sleep. Your body does not move at all and it's tough for anything to wake you. This stage lasts for about a quarter of your sleep time.

Your heart and respiratory functions slow down and you may also dream.

Stage 5: This is called the REM stage, where you are completely relaxed although your eyes move a lot. In this stage, your brain is working to rejuvenate itself and get rid of toxins.

For newborns and babies, these steps are different, as we will see later.

Sleep Hygiene

Like personal hygiene, sleep hygiene is the clinical term for our sleep habits, good or bad.

Good sleep hygiene involves many factors, including structured bedtime hours, relaxing pre-bedtime routines, sleep-promoting foods, and bedroom environment. It's simply a set of good habits and environmental changes geared towards promoting healthy sleep.

Teaching your baby good, lifelong sleep hygiene is what this book is all about.

Why Sleep Training is Important for Your Baby

A large volume of research conducted in the field of newborn and baby sleep has made some remarkable findings - all of which further confirms the importance of baby sleep training.

Here are some ways that good sleep hygiene will benefit your child:

- Children who are trained as babies to develop good sleep habits have higher cognitive abilities. They were also found to receive higher scores on science and math tests. This means that if you start early, you're setting your child up for academic success!

- When you teach your baby effective sleeping skills, he will be less likely to develop ADHD, ADD, and other cognitive disorders.

- Babies who are taught good sleeping habits have a calmer disposition, are friendlier with strangers, and more adaptable in general. This means that early sleep training can spare you lots of temper tantrums!

- Parents who get good rest can bond with their babies better, which is the whole aim of happy parenting.

- There's a strong correlation between sleep and a baby's development. Babies trained to sleep well develop faster and are healthier, while those with poor sleep habits are likely to be frail, sickly, and irritable.

These are just some of the reasons why training your baby to sleep will pay on every level. Plus, they are backed by science!

10 Facts About Baby Sleep

1. A newborn's light sleep and frequent waking during the night is an instinctive response. He has been programmed by Mother Nature to demand sustenance every few hours, especially in the first months of growth and development.

2. Newborns alternate between light sleep and deep sleep every hour or so. This is why they tend to wake up often during the night when they're in the stage of light REM sleep. The key is to teach them to go back to sleep on their own.

3. Why do babies fall asleep faster when they're rocked? Rocking imitates the feeling of being in the womb! Another study has suggested that this is the reason children love swings as well.

4. Adults have 5 sleep stages but babies have just two: deep non-REM sleep and light REM sleep. They rotate between these two stages for the first few months of their lives.

5. There's a reason for babies' light sleep. During this stage of REM rest, the baby's brain is active and blood flow to this area increases, promoting growth and development.

6. Babies sleep a lot, although exhausted parents will call you a liar to your face if you suggest this! But while newborns sleep for up to 18 hours a day, they also wake up frequently, which gives the impression that they are sleepless creatures.

7. Babies who sleep in a darkened room are better able to regulate their circadian rhythm (sleep/wake cycle) as they learn to distinguish between day and night.

8. Closed eyes don't mean your baby's fast asleep. It takes a baby up to 20 minutes to move from a light sleep stage into a deep sleep stage.

9. Contrary to what many parents think, a baby who naps often during the day will not keep you up during the night. A well-rested baby sleeps more soundly at night.

10. Leaving a screaming baby to exhaust himself to sleep can affect brain development and emotional growth. This is because the baby's distress raises cortisol (stress hormone) levels in the baby's body. This can have very negative effects in the long-term. It angers and stuns me that some parents even have the heart to put their baby through this.

Some of these facts you may already know, while others might come as a surprise. The bottom line is this: it's worth your time and effort to train your precious one to get the best possible sleep. The result will be a healthier, happier baby, and healthier, happier parents!

CHAPTER 2

NEWBORN AND BABY SLEEP - WHAT TO EXPECT

A
t last, the ordeal of the birth is over and you are back home with the tiny new addition to your family. For first-time parents, those early weeks will be a whirlwind of conflicting emotions; euphoria, fear, confusion, excitement, and anxiety. This applies to veteran parents as well, although usually to a lesser extent because they more or less know what to expect.

Knowing what you can expect with regards to your newborn's sleep will ease your mind and reassure you that everything is normal in that area. During those first few weeks though, be prepared for a lot of sleep deprivation until your newborn's sleep training kicks in.

Newborn Sleep - Birth to 8 Weeks

I
n the first 8 weeks of life, your newborn will display the following sleep patterns:

▓ Your newborn thinks that day is night and vice-versa! The explanation is simple: Mommy's movement during her pregnancy. As you went about your activities during the day, your movement soothed and rocked the baby to sleep in your womb, and he slept during the day. When you went to bed at night and the rocking movement stopped, your baby would wake up. You may even have noticed that the baby tended to kick and move more when you were resting. What fascinating little beings babies are!

▦ As I mentioned earlier, newborns sleep a lot! Your next question will be one of incredulity: then why is he keeping us up all night? Babies tend to sleep in chunks. Although they require loads of sleep during this early period, they're also programmed to wake up often to be fed. This is why parents get the impression that their baby hardly sleeps.

▦ A typical newborn will sleep between 16-18 hours a day. Some sleep up to 20 hours a day. The early weeks are a cycle of sleeping, waking up to nurse, and soiling diapers. So, be patient and don't despair. There will come a time when your baby will sleep through the night.

▦ A newborn's sleep pattern is unpredictable during the first 8 weeks due to his sleep cycle. Whereas we transition through 5 various stages that allow us to sleep for 8 hours nightly, a newborn alternates between two stages: light sleep and deep sleep. Both cycles are short, and he will wake up to be nursed during the light sleep cycle. When he goes back to sleep, he will remain in a light stage for about 30 minutes, then transition into a deep sleep, and so on.

The Phases of Newborn Sleep

Since your newborn will not have a regular sleep cycle, he may sleep longer some days and stay up longer on others. But there are phases in his sleep/wake pattern that you can expect to observe.

1. **Quiet phase**

   This is the phase immediately after your baby wakes up. He will remain still and quiet for a time and will also be alert. He may respond to sounds and movement. During this phase, your newborn is taking in his new environment.

2. **Crying phase**

   The baby will start to fidget and then to cry, balling his fists and kicking his legs. In this phase, the baby shouldn't be left to become too agitated. It's okay to cradle him or wrap him snugly in a blanket to calm him down. Ideally, when you notice your baby starts to become restless, you should feed him before he starts crying.

3. **Sleep readiness phase**

   After feeding and changing the baby, he may return

to the quiet/alert phase again, and will show signs of sleepiness. These include fussiness, yawning, rubbing his eyes, or crying.

4. **Sleep phase**
   The baby then falls asleep again and the cycle repeats itself every two to three hours.

First 8 Weeks

Every baby is different when it comes to sleep, but these are the general patterns you should expect to see in the first 8 weeks.

During this time, newborns are unable to distinguish between day or night, or form their sleep patterns. Understanding some of the signs such as sleep readiness can help you create a healthy and safe sleep routine for your baby.

Baby Sleep: 2-12 Months

From the second month up to his first year, your baby's sleep patterns will begin to change. Nothing dramatic, but you'll notice a gradual, steady change that indicates that your child is healthy and settling into a normal sleep routine.

The good news is that your baby will begin to sleep longer during the night and stay awake longer during the day. You'll experience the wonderful joy of bonding and interacting with your precious child on a deeper level as he begins to discover his new world. Here's what to expect:

2-3 Months

▦ Your baby still needs to sleep for about 14-16 hours of the day.

▦ Your baby will start to show more settled sleep patterns for both day and night sleep. He'll stay asleep a little longer during the night. If, for example, he was waking up every 2-3 hours during the night, he may now begin sleeping for 4-5 hour intervals during the night.

▦ At 3 months, the baby's sleep cycle changes and he spends longer times in deep sleep.

3-6 Months

▦ Your baby still needs between 14-16 hours of sleep out of 24.

▦ Night sleep will gradually increase until the baby sleeps for up to 6 hours a night by the time he is around 6 months old.

His daytime sleep will decrease, and he'll need 2-3 naps (of 1-2 hours' duration) during the day.

6-12 Months

There are two important developments to be aware of at this stage: At six months and upwards, an amazing change takes place. Baby is embarking on an exciting, thrilling adventure - he's discovering a whole new world filled with fascinating things to explore! To keep up with all the excitement, he develops two awesome abilities:

1. Your little one develops the ability to keep himself awake! Who needs sleep when so many exciting things are waiting to be discovered, and when he is developing new skills and abilities to explore them? You can therefore expect settling to be more difficult from 6 months on, especially when your baby starts crawling and becoming more active.

2. Babies begin to experience separation anxiety. They are now able to understand that even when Mommy and Daddy are not in the room, they're somewhere nearby.

This is an amazing development because babies begin to grasp that even when things can't be seen, they're still there. You can therefore expect your baby to fuss or cry in order to draw you back to his side.

Also, you can expect the following:

▓ Your baby will still need a lot of sleep during this important phase of growth and development. Babies will typically sleep 15-16 hours a day.

▓ Your baby will also sleep longer during the night and will need less time to fall asleep.

▓ The baby's sleep cycle begins to mature into that of an adult, which means that he will wake up less often during the night.

▓ Daytime sleep becomes less frequent and most babies typically require 1-2 naps lasting 1-2 hours.

Takeaways

K nowing what to expect during the first 12 months should ease your mind about your baby developing and behaving normally. Again, these developments are not set in stone, as every baby is different. For some, the developments will be slower while for others they will be faster. As long as your child's sleep patterns and behavior falls somewhere within the ranges discussed here, everything's fine. Now that you know more about a baby's sleep patterns during the first year, observe your baby and note his specific cycle of sleep. This will help you customize the perfect sleep routine that will promote your child's optimum health and wellbeing, and preserve your sanity during this hectic and exciting time.

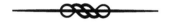

CHAPTER 3

SETTLING TECHNIQUES & ROUTINES

B efore your baby can drift off into sound, restful sleep, he needs to be "settled", or soothed and relaxed. Settling is also the foundation of a good sleep routine, so it's good to introduce a consistent settling routine as soon as your baby's born. It gently teaches your baby to recognize that it's beddy-bye time and relate the feeling of comfort and security to sleep.

Signs of Tiredness

S igns of tiredness in your child are your cue to step in and settle him as soon as possible. Sometimes, even if you have a sleep schedule in place, your baby may need to be put to bed earlier or take a short nap during the day. This is especially true when he starts crawling and becoming more active, which tends to result in overexerting his little body.

Remember, a well-rested baby sleeps better, so if you observe the signs, initiate your settling routine. Try not to let your baby become overtired because this will make it harder to settle him and get him to fall asleep.

When to Start Looking for Signs of Tiredness

Depending on your child's age, he will begin to show tiredness signs after a certain time since his last sleep.

These timings are as follows:

Newborns up to 8 weeks	1 and 1/2 hours after waking up
3-6 months	1 and 1/2 to 3 hours after waking up
6-12 months	2-3 hours after waking up
12-18 months	A morning or afternoon nap is sufficient

Signs of Tiredness in Newborns

Newborns will start to display signs of tiredness not too long after they wake up, typically within an hour or so. You might see some of the following tired signs:

- Clenched fists

- Sucking on the fingers

- Yawning

- Closed or fluttering eyes

- Jerking of arms and legs or kicking

- Pulling his ears

- Shut eyes

- Fluttering eyes

- Cranky, sporadic crying

- Crossed eyes – don't panic, it's normal!

Signs of Tiredness in Babies and Toddlers

When it comes to recognizing the first symptoms of tiredness in babies and toddlers, some of the common signs are:

- Grumpiness

- Crying for attention

- Temper tantrums

- Frowning or looking distressed

- Fussiness with food

- Hyperactivity

- Refusal to go to bed

Learn to identify your child's tiredness signals and put him to bed without delay, otherwise, settling him may become a real ordeal.

Note: A baby displays all of these signs if he's hungry as well. As a parent, you will be able to distinguish when your child's crank is because he's hungry or because he's tired, depending on your feeding and bedtime routine.

Settling Techniques to Help Your Baby Sleep: Newborns - 12 months

By establishing a settling routine from the very first day that you bring your newborn home, you are instilling an invaluable skill. During his first year. Your baby will gradually learn to self-settle and fall asleep on his own with minimum fuss.

Again, this is a personalized process. Some babies may learn to self-settle after a few months while for others, the process will be slower.

Why a Settling Routine is Important

Settling routines in children are important for many reasons, especially when it comes to sleeping. For example:

1. Remember, your newborn is adjusting to a new world after living in the warm, safe home of Mommy's womb. Physical touch, soothing sounds, and closeness are essential to calming and comforting him.

2. Your baby will quickly adapt and respond to settling when you do it consistently. When you respond to his tiredness signs by settling, he will be soothed quickly, allowing him   to get the rest he needs.

3. A consistent settling routine is the first step in helping your child develop good sleep habits.

The following are some settling options to choose from.

Newborn - 6 Months

Arm Settling

This is ideal for the first month or two. Cuddle your baby gently in your arms while rocking or stroking him softly. You can also sing to him if you want. When he falls asleep, continue with the settling process for a few minutes then lay him gently in his crib.

Hand Settling

Cuddle your baby and talk to him softly for a few moments as you walk to his sleeping space. Gently place him in his crib. Stroke him gently while making soothing sounds until he falls asleep.

Patting Technique

Lay your baby on his side facing away from you. Pat him softly on the thigh or bottom with gentle, rhythmic movements. You can also speak in a soothing voice, hum, or sing to him until he falls asleep.

This technique can be done in two ways. You can settle him as he lies on your lap, or you can use this technique as he lies in his crib. When he falls asleep, turn him gently onto his back and leave the room. Try both and see which one settles your baby faster.

6-12 Months

Hand Settling

This is the same as the hand settling technique for newborns, except that in this case, you leave the room before the baby falls asleep. If he starts crying, repeat the process.

Distance Settling

Get your baby ready for bed and place him in his crib with a goodnight kiss and a little cuddle. Sit in a nearby chair where the child can see you. Close your eyes as if you are sleeping.

If he stays awake or starts to fuss, make little "Shhh" sounds to comfort him. If he starts crying, go to his crib and stroke him for a few moments with soothing sounds, but don't pick him up. When the baby calms down, go back to your chair.

As your baby learns to fall asleep with this technique, the next stage is to leave the room after settling him in his crib.

When Your Baby Won't Settle

Hunger, thirst, fear, a wet/soiled diaper, or feeling too hot/cold can keep your baby crying and fussing. Identify what the problem is and resolve it with the following tips.

░ Give him a "top-up" feed if you think he's still hungry. This, along with you cradling him as he nurses, should do the trick.

░ Swaddling: This is an age-old technique used for keeping babies from fussing. You simply wrap your baby snugly to restrict involuntary movement, which can calm a distressed or overtired baby.

░ Use a light cotton wrap such as a small sheet. Keeping the baby's arms at waist level, wrap him snugly but not too tightly; just enough to keep him from flailing his arms and legs. Cuddle your baby or rock him until he settles.

░ Try giving your baby some boiled and cooled water in case he's thirsty.

░ If the weather's nice, take the baby outside for a while. This is a technique that usually works well for super-cranky, overtired babies.

░ Make sure it's not colic. Colic is a common problem that newborns suffer from. The exact cause is unknown although many medical experts believe that it's caused by pain due to gas in the baby's stomach. If your baby is healthy but cries nonstop, see your pediatrician. There are many natural and safe medicines to alleviate the baby's discomfort. Colic may make your settling routine more difficult, but babies do outgrow it over time.

If all attempts to quieten your baby fail, there could be a more serious underlying issue. He could be in pain or coming down with something. If this is the case, you will need to contact your pediatrician immediately.

Useful Settling tips

Pay Attention to How You're Feeling

If your baby is taking too long to settle, you may start getting angry or frustrated. Your patting or stroking may unconsciously become rougher and less rhythmic, which will make things worse. Also, if you're singing or making shushing sounds, pay attention that your voice doesn't become loud or impatient.

It's Okay to Use a Pacifier

As long as it's not in your infant's mouth 24/7, it's perfectly fine to use a pacifier as a settling aid, especially if your baby takes longer to fall asleep. This usually works well for "tough" babies. Make sure to gently remove the pacifier as soon as the baby falls asleep.

Master the Art of Patting

That's right, patting is an art! It has to be "just so" for your baby to fall asleep. Soft, gentle, and rhythmic is the recipe for success. If you drift off and daydream as you're settling your baby and lose the rhythm, the baby will start to fret. Try it and see for yourself.

A great idea is to play some soft music and pat your baby along to the beat so that you keep a consistent rhythm. With practice, you'll soon become a pro, with or without music!

Play Music

Most babies adore music. Try playing some soft music as you settle to help your baby drift off peacefully. If you choose to do this, you'll notice that over time, your baby will develop a preference for a specific song!

Read to Your Baby

This is a good way to settle some babies from 6 months and upwards and is a good introduction to the traditional bedtime story. Read something to your baby in a soft voice as he lies in his crib. The words will be gibberish to him but the soft tone and inflections in your voice will soothe and calm him.

Experiment With Settling Techniques

Try each of the techniques discussed above to discover which one your baby responds to best. Some babies like to be petted but not rocked. Some like to be rocked but not stroked. Some will fall asleep the first time you leave the room; others will need to be comforted longer. It's your job to find the perfect balance that works with your little one's needs.

Note: Once you find the best technique, stick to it. Consistency is key to settling techniques.

Takeaways

Settling techniques are essential for instilling good sleep hygiene in your baby, and making life a lot easier for parents. The earlier your baby learns to settle and fall asleep, the easier it will be for you to create a healthy sleep routine that promotes his growth, development, and wellbeing. Your labor of love is to lay the groundwork for a healthy, happy, wonderful child.

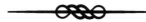

CHAPTER 4

CREATING THE PERFECT SLEEP ROUTINE

N ow, it's time to learn how to set your baby up for life with good sleep habits. It starts with creating an effective sleep routine.

Sleep disorders and poor sleep issues are becoming more prevalent today as our lives become more hectic and stressful. Usually, the roots of these problems lie in poor sleep hygiene during childhood. By instilling sound sleep habits in your baby, you're giving him a head start to a healthy, successful, productive life. The bonus is that you will have significantly less stress and hassle during the early years of parenting.

The Essentials of a Good Bedtime Routine

T here's no specific routine that works better than another. An ideal bedtime routine is one that is tailored to your baby's sleep patterns and preferences and that suits your family's needs. However, it should fall within the following framework:

- Bedtime routines need to be structured and consistent, because fixed hours and activities allow your baby to develop healthy sleep habits. Babies may not show it, but they love structure and consistency. It gives them a sense of stability and security in a new and sometimes overwhelming environment.

- Nap and bedtime schedules should be organized around your family's schedule so that you can stay consistent.

- Sleep rituals should create a relaxing transition from the bustle and activity of the day to a quiet, restful night. They should be enjoyed by you and your child and as a peaceful time of closeness and bonding. Your child must make this association early on.

- Sleep routines should be implemented gradually and with patience. Your baby should slowly learn to associate sleep with relaxation, pleasurable feelings, and love. Trying to force it on him too quickly will create very negative associations that can affect him for the rest of his life.

When to Start a Sleep Routine

A short bedtime routine can be initiated starting at 8 weeks. Earlier than that is not very realistic. Remember, both you and your baby need time to adjust. Baby needs time to take in his new environment, and you need time to adapt your life around his needs and familiarize yourself with his sleeping patterns.

For the first 8 weeks, ease your baby into a structured sleep routine by using the settling techniques discussed in the previous chapter. After that, you can start a short sleep routine and gradually build upon it.

Infant Sleep Routines: 8 Weeks – 12 Months

You can start sleep routines 45-30 minutes before bedtime. 30 minutes might be better for babies under 6 months, while a 45-minute routine that incorporates some play or story-telling may work better when your baby passes the 6-month milestone.

You should incorporate two or three of the following activities:

- **Top-up feed -** or light snacks such as baby applesauce or strained bananas if your baby is eating. If you make this the first step of your bedtime routine, make sure your baby eats a little less on the prior feed. If your baby is just not hungry, don't force him, just carry on with the other steps of the routine.

- **Warm bath -** nothing soothes a baby like a warm bath with mild chamomile soap. Some babies may cry while they are being bathed but when they're dried, dressed, and snuggled, they will very quickly settle down and become drowsy. Please note that experts do not recommend bathing an infant every day as this will dry out their skin. You can consider giving your baby a warm bath twice weekly and replace this step with a baby massage on the other nights of the week. This is fine and your baby will grow accustomed to both routines as a "sleep signal."

- **Oral hygiene -** if your baby has cut some teeth, brush them very gently with a soft, moist toothbrush but no toothpaste, while making fun, encouraging sounds. Next, wipe his gums with a moist washcloth. If your baby hasn't cut his teeth yet, wipe his gums gently for a few moments while making soothing sounds.

- **Baby massage -** research has found that infant massage has many benefits for a baby's health, in addition to being a soothing pre-bedtime technique. There's a wide variety of coaching videos on YouTube if you'd like to learn how it's done in more detail. Here's a good example: http://bit.ly/babymassagetips

- **Play or sing lullabies -** lullabies have been a bedtime staple for centuries. Today, technology and science have come together to provide you with hundreds of downloadable lullabies specifically designed to soothe your baby and put him in the mood for sleep. You can start playing them as soon as you start the sleep routine so that the baby can enjoy them as he is being bathed, massaged, or fed.

■ **Good night snuggles and cuddles** - this is the last step in your routine. Cuddle and kiss your baby, place him in his crib and say a soft goodnight.

■ **Play white noise -** white noise is a combination of different frequencies that create a soothing hum or buzz which blocks out the sounds of the external environment. A ceiling fan, humming refrigerator, or television turned down low are good examples. Studies have found that white noise mimics the sounds inside a mother's womb. Contrary to what we may think, it's not silent in there. There's that "whoosh" of fluid as the baby moves, as well as the various sounds of Mommy's vital functions, like her heartbeat, growling stomach, and various digestion noises. These sounds are familiar and calming for the baby. White noise apps that you can play on a phone or tablet are widely available, so you may want to check them out at the App Store or Google Play Store.

Short Story

I know a dad who worked as an audio engineer. Before his baby was born, he recorded the sounds inside his wife's womb. He made a loop of the recording and placed a playback device under his baby son's crib. He reported that it worked like a charm! The parents never had any trouble getting their baby to fall asleep.

If you're lucky enough to be reading this book before your baby's birth, it could be a great and fun idea to try. I love it! I'm not sure about the technicalities of how it's done but with so many tech wizards all around us, it should be easy to find someone who can help you do this.

You can also consider apps that play nature sounds such as falling rain, ocean waves, or chirping birds. These are all options to experiment with to test your baby's preferences.

Building on Baby's Sleep Routine

As your baby grows, you can add or make changes to his bedtime ritual. This could include a short playtime in the bath, helping him brush his teeth and put on pajamas, reading stories, playing with his favorite stuffed toy, and so on. All of this will fall into place as you and your baby discover his likes and dislikes together. As long as you have a consistent and structured sleep routine in place, you already have a solid foundation to build on.

Tips for a More Effective Sleep Routine

- **Create the right atmosphere -** we'll discuss this in more detail in a later chapter, but these are the basics you need to do right before you start your sleep routine:

A. Dim the lights or close the curtains. This is important for helping your baby develop his circadian rhythm, allowing him to start learning to differentiate between day and night, and to associate nighttime with sleep.

B. Quiet is important as well, so make sure there are no distractions like a TV or ringing cell phones.

Adjust as necessary - at the beginning, your baby's sleep may respond more to white noise or lullabies. As he grows older, you can stick to reading a bedtime story or a more elaborate bath time ritual. He may require more snuggling and cuddling, or a short massage. You get the idea. Just go with the flow and make adjustments as needed.

The baby should always sleep in the same place - your infant must learn to associate a designated place with sleeping - namely, his crib. Switching sleeping places often, say from playpen to pram to crib, can be a little confusing for your baby. Plus, if he develops a preference for sleeping in his stroller, you've got a problem! It's okay to settle a newborn in a stroller but once he's older, he needs to fall asleep in his crib.

Note: This applies to naps as well. Your baby should learn to do all of his sleeping in his crib.

▦ **Create an abbreviated naptime routine -** use an association that your baby is already familiar with, such as white noise or a lullaby, to initiate a short nap time routine. This will foster your baby's sleep habits further as well as help him sleep more restfully.

▦ **Be flexible when necessary -** as your baby grows, he will become more active, which means that some days, he will overexert himself in play and discovery. Be on the alert for tiredness signs and start your sleep routine immediately if you spot them. Even if it's an hour before his regular bedtime or if he needs an extra nap, ditch the schedule for that day and put your baby to sleep.

▦ **Help your baby recognize day and night -** you want your baby to develop a balanced circadian rhythm as soon as possible. This means you need to help him differentiate between day and night. During the day, let in as much light as possible into the house. You can even keep the lights on during the day if you don't get much sunlight. Bustle around energetically and make as much noise as you want to. This signals to your child that daytime is for work, play, and activity. In the evening, close the curtains and dim the light, make as little noise as possible. Move more slowly to teach your baby that nighttime is for quiet, calm, and sleep.

▨ **Be patient and firm** - the goal of an effective sleep routine is to help your baby fall asleep on his own. Once you have reached the stage where you place him in his crib, don't back down! It may take repeated settling, soothing, and going in and out of the room. You may be tempted to just pick him up and rock him to sleep. My best advice, exhausted and frustrated as you may be, is don't give in. Be patient and firm. Your baby is finally going to fall asleep and it will get a little easier each time.

Sample Bedtime Routine

Here is a sample routine that should take no more than 35 - 40 minutes. It will give you a better idea of how to proceed.

35 – 40 minutes before sleep

• Dim the lights, turn off TV and cell phones, turn on lullabies/ white noise/ nature sounds. Keep your movement slow and quiet.

• Bath your baby/ baby massage or change his diaper and top off with baby lotion or baby powder.

• Give a top-off feed if needed.

• Brush teeth or wipe gums

15-20 minutes before bed

• Read a story while snuggling or simply cradle your baby lovingly.

5 minutes before sleep

• As your baby gets drowsy, place him in his crib, soothe him and say goodnight. If the baby is already in his crib during the story reading, pat him gently as he falls asleep and leave the room.

Takeaways

No sleep routine is set in stone. There's just no one-size-fits-all that parents can simply copy and paste. Every sleep routine is individual to a baby's preferences, and it's up to you to discover what they are and create a customized plan that fits into the basic framework discussed here. It will take patience and effort because habits take time to form. But always remember that you are giving your child something invaluable: great sleep associations and habits that will serve him well throughout his lifetime.

CHAPTER 5

NIGHT WEANING AND PHASING OUT NIGHT FEEDS

ew parents are united around a single wish and a seemingly impossible dream: to sleep through the night! This of course is only possible if their baby sleeps through the night. Don't despair! With a good sleep routine in place, you will slowly but surely progress towards that glorious day when you can sleep for a full 6, 7, or even 8 hours.

Here's some good news; you can accelerate the process and bring that day closer by helping your baby make a smooth transition into night weaning.

What is Night Weaning?

ust as the term implies, it means weaning your child from night feeds so that he gradually learns to sleep for more hours during the night and eventually, the whole night through. A word of warning here: it's not easy. If you think settling your baby is hard, you haven't tried night weaning. I'm not trying to discourage you by any means, but I do advise you to be prepared for a rough ride for a couple of weeks. However, parents who have tried it report that it's well worth the effort.

Many parents are now opting for night weaning because those extra few hours of sleep (especially for working parents) are priceless.

Night weaning is not mandatory for good sleep training. It's a decision that has more to do with the parents' needs than the baby's. Your baby is going to sleep through the night sooner or later on his own. With night weaning, you are speeding up the process to get some much-needed rest.

Parents who have a lot of family support, such as grandparents coming on board to share night duty, may not need to wean their baby and are able to just let things proceed naturally. This is common in eastern cultures where parents or in-laws may live with the parents and play an active role in taking care of the baby.

When Can Parents Begin Night Weaning?

The short answer is when your baby's ready but not before 4 months. 4-6 months is the age recommended by pediatricians but again, it depends on the baby. If he's healthy and eating well throughout the day, it is possible to start night weaning as early as 4 months. A well-fed baby will typically wake up during the night out of habit rather than hunger. The trick is to settle the baby without feeding him until he goes back to sleep.

At 4-6 months, your baby will be introduced to solid food and is considered ready for night weaning.

If you feel your baby is ready, consult your pediatrician and never start night weaning on your own. The pediatrician will confirm whether it's okay based on your baby's growth.

Note: Never start night weaning when your baby is teething.

Expert Opinions

What do the experts tell us about night weaning?

Pediatrician William Sears stresses that night feedings are important for parent/child bonding and advises parents not to cut out night feedings completely until the child is ready to sleep through the night on his own.

Other pediatricians like Richard Ferber suggest that frequent night feedings can cause digestive problems that cause the baby to wake up even more frequently during the night. He recommends night weaning as a way to avoid these problems.

Some experts say that doing it in one go and cutting out all night feeds is possible. Personally, and I hope you'll agree, I think it's too harrowing a process to put yourself and your baby through. You don't need to be an expert to see that this is plain common sense.

Remember, we're trying to create positive associations with sleep. 4 or 5 horrible nights of your baby screaming through the night (which is approximately how long it takes to cut out night feedings in one go) will create anything but a positive association. And really, what parent has the heart to do this when it's not imperative?

So, as you can see, there is no consensus from experts around whether parents should night wean. Ultimately, this is a decision that you have to make.

The 4 Steps of Night Weaning

1. Increase Day Feeds

Keeping your baby well-fed during the day will decrease his chances of waking up during the night.

Try feeding your baby more food around bedtime, or even their main baby food dinner around bedtime to ensure that his stomach is full of good, warm food.

Increase the amount of formula or breast milk you give your child during the day by an ounce or two. If he is eating baby food, be sure to give him a filling meal in the evening.

2. Go Slow and Gradual

I'm sure you already know that this won't happen overnight. Gradually cut out one feed per night for two or three nights, then reduce by two feeds, and so on. Depending on your baby's response, he should be down to one or two feeds after about 10 days.

When your child wakes up during the no-feed time, settle him as he lies in his crib until he falls asleep. If he's been well fed before bedtime, chances are that he's waking up out of habit.

Don't try and eliminate all the night feedings at once. It will never work and both you and your baby will find it very challenging. Instead, if you're used to getting up four times a night, take it down to three for the first few days.

Shorten feeding times during the night, putting your baby immediately back in his crib after he has nursed.

In a nutshell, night weaning means prolonging the times between feeds and shortening the feeds themselves. Gradually, your baby will begin to respond to the new routine. He will start to learn that nighttime is for sleeping rather than for eating.

3. Patience!

Don't give up! Be flexible when necessary within reason and have patience. You'll probably see some small results in about 3 or 4 days. Give your child time to adjust on his own.

4. Provide a Comfort Source

Babies sometimes wake up because they want to be cuddled and comforted. When you are night weaning, you can also teach your baby to comfort himself if he wakes up. Place a favorite stuffed toy beside him that he can cuddle up with instead of you when he wakes up. Let him hold the toy and play with it before bedtime so that learns to make the association. A small snuggly blanket can also help your baby self-settle, just remember that many objects inside the crib may compromise the baby safety when he sleeps.

What to Expect

You'll see the first small transition in about 3-4 days as your baby begins to adjust to going without one feed. The whole process will take about a week to a week and a half. Just be prepared for a lot of crying and settling during the first few days.

Most babies can be night weaned but, in the rare case that your little one does not adjust to the changes, it may be more trouble than it's worth. You may want to consider ditching the night weaning and going back to your normal routine.

Takeaways

Night weaning is not mandatory and ultimately, the decision comes down to you. Just remember to increase feedings during the day to ensure that your baby is getting all the nutrients and calories he needs. Remember to consult your pediatrician even if you feel your baby is ready for night weaning, and finally, be patient!

Sleep-deprived parents may opt for night weaning to maintain their wellbeing, so if you feel a few extra hours of sleep are worth the effort of night weaning your baby, go for it!

CHAPTER 6

THE PERFECT SLEEP ENVIRONMENT FOR THE BABY

N ow, it's time to add the next pillar to the ideal sleep routine for your baby. You want to create the most calming, cozy, inviting environment that helps your baby drift off into sound sleep and sweet dreams.

Creating the perfect sleep environment is possible regardless of your living conditions. Any changes you may have to make are minimal and cost-effective. Once in place, the following components will suit any child from birth well into his early years. These components are backed by science and all work together to promote quality sleep.

Baby's Crib

S ome thought should go into your baby's crib since it will be his primary sleep companion for quite some time. Always look for quality over cost as this is a sound investment to make in return for your baby's comfort and safety. The following chapter will discuss baby sleep safety in more detail.

░ Make sure the crib is marked with the following code: BSEN-716-2-2008. This means the cot complies with baby safety regulations and standards.

░ The mattress should be waterproof, thin, and firm.

░ Make sure the bars are at a proper distance and don't allow for the baby's head to get through.

░ The crib should be deep enough so that when your baby reaches the stage where he is able to pull himself up to a standing position, the bar is at the neck or high waist level.

░ Ideally, avoid cribs with cutouts to avoid the baby's arm getting stuck.

░ Test the mattress fit to make sure it fits snugly into the crib contours and that there are no gaps where the baby's arms or legs can get stuck.

Room Temperature

Cooler is better. This may come as a surprise to you and you're not alone. Many parents tend to bundle up their babies snugly for sleep and turn up the room temperature, thinking that warmth will help the baby sleep better. It's not surprising that a lot of parents are under this misconception. Babies are such tiny, fragile creatures that it makes sense to assume they need to be kept warm and toasty.

However, science tells us that the opposite is true. During the day, our internal temperature peaks, then begins to go down with the onset of evening. This is the natural body temperature cycle of humans. During night sleep, the body temperature is at its lowest. Nature has designed us to sleep better when our body temperatures are lower.

If your baby's room is too warm, your baby will not fall asleep as fast. His body will expend a lot of energy to regulate his body temperature to one that is optimal for sleep. But if the room matches the baby's inner temperature, he will quickly drift off to sleep and sleep more soundly. Strange, but true!

So, what's the ideal temperature for your baby's room? According to the experts, 67-72 degrees Fahrenheit is ideal. If you are unable to control the temperature in individual rooms of your home, this is a very reasonable temperature for the household and should not be too uncomfortable.

As an additional precaution, note the following signs to understand if your baby's room is too hot or too cold.

▷ **If the baby's room is too hot -** your baby's skin may feel damp or his head might be sweaty. Overheating is one of the major causes that can prevent a child from sleeping well. Lighter sleepwear or turning down the temperature a notch or two will solve the problem.

▷ **If the baby's room is too cold** - your baby's nose and hands may feel cold and the core body area (chest and back) will feel cold to the touch. If this is the case, raise the room temperature by a degree or two or add an extra layer to your baby's clothing.

Sleepwear

Comfort and safety are the top priorities when it comes to choosing your baby's sleepwear. This is especially true for newborns up to 6 months.

- The best sleepwear for babies is one-piece pajamas with built-in booties. You probably wore them yourself!

- Sleepwear should fit snugly but not too tightly. Avoid loose clothing as research has suggested that this could be a contributing factor to SIDS (more about that later).

- Avoid clothing that can ride up over the baby's face or twist around his body. This is why snuggly one-pieces are the best option and will never go out of fashion.

- If the room temperature is within the recommended range, a baby may need a light layer of underclothing such as a onesie.

- You can also consider a baby sleep sack as an extra layer.

- Ideally, sleepwear and sleep sacks should be hoodless.

- Always choose cotton sleepwear for summer and warmer material for winter. Always avoid synthetic material, especially directly against your baby's sensitive skin.

The advice suggested here is perfect for newborns up to the age of six months and even up to one year. For toddlers, slight changes can be made, such as an extra coverlet or blanket, two-piece pajamas, and no baby sack.

If you're a fashion friend and want your baby to be the trendiest sleeper on the block, take a fun break and check out these cool baby pajamas! You'll also find some more helpful hints on the ideal sleepwear for your baby.

▷ http://bit.ly/babypajamasreview

Lighting

This may come as another surprise to you but your baby's room should be like Batman's cave - as dark as possible. For some reason, parents think babies are afraid of the dark. And yet, they managed to live quite comfortably in the pitch darkness of Mommy's womb. Babies are not afraid of the dark. In fact, the sooner your newborn adapts to a dark room, the fewer problems you will have in the future, as he may develop a fear of the dark. You can see this in some grown adults who are unable to sleep in a darkened room. This probably goes back to their childhood sleep training.

A volume of research studies has confirmed that a dark environment is vital to a baby's sleep for several reasons:

- Darkness helps a baby associate darkness and nighttime with sleep.

- Sleep quality is better in darkness.

- Exposure to light during sleep can alter a baby's internal body clock and sleep rhythm.

- Darkness promotes the production of melatonin, commonly known as the "sleep hormone". Our body begins producing more melatonin as night sets in to prepare us for rest. It promotes drowsiness, relaxes the muscles, and induces yawning. Light slows down melatonin production, whereas a darkened room helps your baby's body continue producing the sleep-inducing hormone throughout the night, allowing him to sleep more soundly.

Even light filtering in from the street or nightlights can slow down melatonin production so ideally, your baby's room should be completely dark. You may want to consider blackout curtains or a very small night light at a distance from the baby's crib.

Bedding

During the first year of his life, your baby is going to spend a large part of his time sleeping, so the right bedding is important for his maximum comfort.

Your little one's crib needs to be complemented with suitable bedding. When selecting these items, you'll be charmed by the huge variety of pretty colors and super-cute prints. So, have a blast selecting your baby's bedding but keep the following tips in mind:

- Sheets and crib liners should be made of natural fabric and suitable for the weather.

- All bedding should be machine-washable and easy to maintain.

- Always use fitted sheets.

- If you are going to use a baby sack, you may be tempted to buy a larger one that will accommodate your baby's growth. But a baby sack needs to be a snug fit for two reasons. Firstly, it gives your baby a sense of being swaddled, which promotes comfort and sleep. Secondly, it prevents your baby from wriggling or slipping down into it.

- 100% cotton is the way to go. A mix of polyester and cotton is not a good option, as it is sometimes sprayed with formaldehyde to prevent wrinkling. "Green" baby linen is made from the finest, silky-soft cotton that is organically treated. It also lasts for ages, so if you're planning on more additions to your family, it could be a better investment in the long run.

- "Green" bedding such as comforters, pillows and blankets may be more expensive but it's made of healthy, natural fibers that are safe for your baby. It can also take a lot of wear and tear and lasts longer. Again, these items could be a more cost-effective investment in the long run.

- Avoid comforters and crib bumpers stuffed with polyester. A healthier choice is a comforter filled with shredded cotton, wool, or rubber. To be honest, they won't stay as fluffy for long, but they are healthier. Having said that, polyester comforters and crib bumpers won't kill your baby. They come in much prettier colors and patterns so if that adorable teddy bear comforter is calling your baby's name, go for it!

Note: when it comes to your baby's crib, use your good sense and always remember "less is more." Many of these thing may compromise the baby safety!

Noise

Your baby needs quiet to sleep well. Loud noises will keep him overstimulated and alert, so always try to make the evening a quieter time throughout the house. This doesn't mean you need to speak in whispers and tiptoe around all night, only until the baby is asleep. You can then resume your normal routine. When starting your baby's bedtime routine, make sure the house is quiet except for lullabies or white noise playing softly. The TV should be turned down low and cell phones should be on silent.

Your baby's room should be in a quiet part of the house if possible. If you live on a noisy street, don't worry. White noise is the answer. Simply play white noise in your baby's room to block out the traffic outside. If possible, consider moving your baby's nursery to a part of the house that is farther away from the street.

More Tips for an Ideal Baby Sleep Environment

▨ Use a fan on extra-hot days to circulate the air and keep your baby cool. Air conditioning is a bad idea. The fan should not be directed full on the baby, but at an angle that creates a cool breeze. Fans are also a great source of white noise, so that's a bonus.

▨ Create a comfortable space for yourself in the nursery. After all, you're going to spend a lot of time there! Have a rocking chair with a comfortable cushion or an easy chair with a footrest where you can relax as you nurse or settle your baby, or even nap a bit as he's napping.

▨ Your baby's room should be well organized with diapers, clothes, and blankets easily accessible for quick night changes and for less hassle overall. Some cribs come with drawers on the bottom where you can neatly store the things you use the most. The last thing you want is to be scrambling around for a diaper in the middle of the night!

▨ Choose soothing colors. Experts recommend painting your baby's room with cool, calming colors like pale blue, green, or yellow. Bright walls and noisy wallpaper can overstimulate your child. Soothing colors are especially important if your baby is going to have a short playtime or story in his room before bedtime.

- Have a minimalist nursery. The minimalist slogan is "less is more" and you would do well to apply this to your baby's nursery. Too many colors and objects can overstimulate your baby and disrupt his sleep. Keep shelves spare and streamlined with everything tucked away in drawers, and consider a big basket for keeping toys out of sight when playtime is over. Also, make sure all cords are hidden away and that the floor is clear.

- Beware of cigarette smoke. If there's a smoker in the house, make sure smoking takes place outdoors from the minute you bring your baby home. If somebody has been smoking, make sure to air your baby's room well before putting him to bed.

- If you live on a noisy, brightly-lit street, custom made blackout shades could solve the problem. They will filter out the light as well as some of the street sounds. If you're on a tight budget, some DIY shades with construction paper will work as well.

Takeaways

Creating an ideal sleeping environment for your baby can be a lot of fun. When you do it smartly with the safe and healthy options discussed here, you can't lose. Kudos on a job that is well done! You're now one step closer to ensuring that your baby enjoys excellent sleep and the sweetest dreams for the rest of his life.

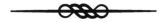

CHAPTER 7

BABY SLEEP SAFETY

Your baby's comfort during sleep needs to go hand in hand with safety. Thankfully, you can provide your little angel with both without compromising on one or the other.

Sleep safety is the third pillar of your baby's sleep routine. All of the pieces discussed in this chapter will fit together to "sleep-proof" your baby and give you the peace of mind that you deserve. Newborns sleep for up to 16 hours a day in the early weeks of life and, therefore, creating a safe sleep space and secure surroundings is highly important.

Sound sleep safety advice combined with a safe sleeping environment dramatically reduces the risk of SIDS (sudden infant death syndrome, or cot death) so it's something that every parent should be well-informed about. Until your baby is 6 months old, the safest place he can sleep is in his crib, preferably in the same room as you or in a room that is next to yours. This is a good arrangement as many parents prefer to have their babies close by in the early months. Your baby should learn to sleep in his crib both at bedtime and naptime.

Sleep-Related Infant Deaths

Okay... let's get the bad stuff out of the way first. I'm going to drag you out of your comfort zone for a little bit. As uncomfortable as the following information may be, every parent needs to know about it. Sleep-related infant deaths are not that common, thank God, but they do occur. In the United States, there are about 3,500 cases per year, commonly labeled "cot deaths". These include SIDS (Sudden Infant Death Syndrome) as well as suffocation and miscellaneous accidents. SIDS is the most common cause of infant cot deaths.

What is SIDS?

The causes of SIDS are as yet unknown. Medical science has been unable to discover the abnormality that causes these deaths and they are classified as deaths by natural causes. Unlike suffocation, which is classified as accidental death, findings do not indicate conclusively that SIDS is caused by asphyxiation. SIDS is still a big mystery to science.

Most SIDS deaths occur in newborns between the ages of 1-4 months. There is no possibility of SIDS occurring after the baby is 12 months old. Parents can rest easy on that point. The great news is that infant sleep-related deaths have gone down over the last 20 years. Again, there's no conclusive evidence as to the reason, but I'd like to think that more awareness about sleep safety by parents plays a role.

11 Tips for Safe Sleeping

1. Put baby to sleep on his back

This is the safest position for healthy babies. Pediatricians strongly urge parents to always place babies on their backs for sleep. Some parents mistakenly think that sleeping on his tummy is more comfortable for the baby but it's quite dangerous. Babies are more likely to die of SUDI (Sudden Unexplained Death in Infancy) including asphyxiation, suffocation, SIDS, and other sleep-related accidents when not sleeping on their backs. Never place your baby to sleep on his stomach or side. At around 4-6 months, your baby will begin to roll over and move around more. Continue placing him on his back at sleep times but allow him to find his preferred sleeping position; it's ok if he rolls over in his sleep. When placing your baby in his crib, place him in the lower part so that his feet are near the bottom.

2. Make sure your baby's head and face are uncovered during sleep

Check that the bedsheet is well tucked in so that it doesn't slip loose and cover the baby's head. Never cover your baby with a blanket but use a sleep sack that leaves his head and face uncovered. Never use headwear of any kind such as a cap or hood. Babies regulate their body temperature through their heads, so your baby's head must be bare so that he doesn't overheat.

3. Eliminate smoking

There's very strong evidence to suggest that exposure to cigarette smoke puts infants at a higher risk of SUDI. This includes smoking during pregnancy. Research also shows that the link between cigarette smoke and SUDI is strong even when parents smoke at a distance from the baby. Ideally, there should be no smoking inside the house at all.

4. Breastfeed your baby

Breastfeeding has been shown to reduce the risk of SIDS and SUDI by more than half, so this is something worth considering. However, if breastfeeding is not a feasible option, make sure you follow the other sleep safety tips and procedures.

5. Keep your baby's crib bare

When it comes to your baby's crib, less is more. Never place pillows, stuffed toys, sleep positioners, bumpers, extra blankets, or comforters in your baby's crib. Nothing should be in the crib except for a snug, fitted sheet - and your baby! Keeping the crib bare eliminates the risk of suffocation and overheating.

6. Phase out swaddling before the baby starts to roll over

Make sure you swaddle your baby properly (don't worry, you'll get the hang of it with practice). Always place a swaddled infant to sleep on his back. When your baby starts trying to roll over, you should have phased out swaddling him, as this can be a strangulation hazard. Swaddling should be completely phased out by the time your baby is rolling over fully at around 3-4 months. If you've been swaddling your baby, start phasing it out gradually at around 2 months to ensure his safety.

7. Use a firm, thin mattress

The safest mattress for your baby is one that is firm, flat, and well-fitted. Make sure that the mattress fits snugly in the crib and that there are no gaps where your baby's head could get stuck. Don't line the mattress with a blanket or add a second mattress. The mattress should be covered only with a thin fitted sheet.

8. Share a room but not a bed

It makes sense to have your newborn in the same room as you. It's more convenient for frequent night feeding, and many parents feel better knowing that their baby is close by. While some experts say it's okay to share a room with your baby during the first year, some parents choose to place him in a separate nursery earlier than that. This is a decision you have to make. Please note that sharing the same room does not mean sharing the same bed. Your baby must have his safely equipped crib in a corner of your room and must learn to sleep separately. In addition to the risks of bed-sharing with parents and the link to SIDS, there's also the possibility that your baby will develop a negative sleep association. It will be harder to train him to sleep independently later on.

9. Don't put your baby to sleep on makeshift bedding, couches, or soft surfaces

Even with supervision, sleeping on a couch is not safe for a baby. Makeshift bedding is also dangerous as the baby could get tangled up in a comforter, wedged between pillows, or struck between the bedding and a wall.

10. Safe sleepwear should be warm but not hot

Overheating has been strongly linked as a cause of SUDI and SIDS. The safest sleepwear for an infant is a one-piece pajama with built-in booties appropriate for the weather and your baby's room temperature. If you feel your baby is too cold, use a sleep sack but monitor him to check for overheating. A flushed face and sweaty head are signs that your baby may be too hot. In this case, you should remove the sleep sack.

11. Try using a pacifier

Believe it or not, pacifiers can help reduce the risk of SIDS. Try giving your baby a pacifier and see if he takes to it. Some babies don't, while breastfed babies tend to sleep better with a pacifier. If the pacifier falls out when your baby is asleep, don't put it back in his mouth. If he is sound asleep with the pacifier in his mouth, gently remove it.

Room Temperature and Ventilation

Always keep in mind that overheating has been associated with SIDS, so monitoring your baby's body and room temperature is a priority. Babies struggle to regulate their body temperature when they're too hot, so the proper room temperature should always be on the cooler side as we discussed earlier. The safety rule is always "cooler is better than hotter".

Co-Sleeping With Baby: How it Reduces SUDI Risk

Y ou may have prepared a nursery for your baby to sleep in, but knowing that sharing a room with your baby reduces the risk of SUDI may cause you to reconsider. It's recommended that you have your baby sleep in your room for the first 6 months, or even 12 months if this is your personal preference. Room sharing allows you to monitor your baby's sounds and check that he is sleeping on his back.

The advantages of having your baby nearby also include the following:

▦ It's more convenient for breastfeeding.

▦ It allows you to respond more quickly to your baby.

▦ You can better monitor your baby for overheating.

▦ Parents have more peace of mind when the baby is sleeping in a separate crib but with them in the same room.

▦ It's easier to train your baby to self-settle and sleep on his own when he feels that you are nearby.

▨ Parents who share a room with their babies report that it creates more bonding and closeness.

Sharing a Bed With Your Baby - What to Consider

Some parents still prefer to have their babies share their bed. Although pediatricians urge against this, it may be a necessity due to cramped living space, or if the mother is breastfeeding, or simply because it gives parents more peace of mind. If you decide to go this route, please be aware of these safety considerations:

▨ Always place the baby on his back to sleep and don't cradle him in your arms.

▨ Make sure you are using a firm, clean mattress and never allow your baby to sleep on a waterbed or any soft surface like a down comforter.

▨ Never allow other children or pets to sleep in the bed.

▨ Your pillows and bedding should be as far away from the baby as possible. Never cover him with the blanket or comforter that you are using.

▨ Make sure the bed is large enough that there is space around your baby.

Your bedding should consist of lightweight blankets. Avoid heavy quilts or comforters.

Do not place the baby on the side of the bed next to a wall. If possible, center your bed so that it is away from the walls.

Always remove your jewelry before going to bed with your baby.

If you're a heavy sleeper, this can be a real danger to your baby. You may roll over on him or throw an arm or leg over his head. In this case, I would strongly urge you not to share a bed with your baby.

Breastfeeding and Bed-Sharing

Breastfeeding is the main reason that mothers prefer to have babies share their bed. Although this is not advisable, it's understandable. You're just so tired and the thought of getting up from a warm bed for endless night feedings is just too overwhelming. If you are breastfeeding your baby in your bed, always use the "cuddle-curl" position. It's likely that you already take this position as it is the most natural and comfortable one. Also, it's the safest for your baby.

The "cuddle-curl" position involves lying on your side, flexing your knees, and placing your arm under and around your baby in a protective "curl". If you fall asleep as you're nursing the baby, your bent legs will prevent you from rolling onto him, and your curled arm provides a protective space. When your baby falls asleep, he will stay on his back with his head turned towards the breast so that's easily accessible. So, if you're breastfeeding, always make sure you do it the best possible way with the cuddle-curl.

Feeding and Sleep Safety

Below are some helpful tips about feeding and sleep safety.

- When breastfeeding or nursing your baby before bed, he will often fall asleep as he's eating. Always make sure to burp him gently before placing him in his crib. Always burp your baby after night feeds as well. This will reduce the chances of gas and excessive vomiting of milk.

- When your baby is eating solid foods, always feed him dinner about 1 to 1.5 hours before bedtime, allowing time for digestion.

- Babies who breastfeed may need a pacifier to fall asleep and that's okay. Research has shown that pacifiers reduce the risk of SIDS. Just make sure to gently remove it after your baby has fallen asleep.

Swaddling and Sleep Safety

M any parents swear by swaddling. They report that when all else fails, a swaddle always helps soothe a baby. Pediatricians agree that swaddling is an effective way to soothe a baby and help him sleep better – if done correctly. A too-loose swaddle could get unwrapped and become a suffocation hazard. If you want to consider swaddling, check with your baby first to see how he responds. While some babies love it, others hate it. So, your baby needs to have the last say here!

Swaddle Your Baby Step-By-Step

Step 1: Use a solid, flat surface such as a changing table or countertop. Spread out the swaddling blanket diagonally in a diamond shape with the top corner pointed above where your baby's head will rest. Fold the top corner downwards by about 6 inches.

Step 2: Lay the baby face-up on the swaddle with his head above the folded top corner. His body should be completely straight from the top to the bottom corners.

Step 3: Keeping the baby's left arm straight, fold the left part of the swaddle over his arm and chest and tuck it firmly under his right side.

Step 4: Bring the bottom part of the blanket up over the baby's body and place it under the first fold. Straighten the baby's arm then fold the right side of the blanket over his chest, tucking it into the left side.

Step 5: Secure the swaddle by twisting the bottom part lightly and tucking it under your baby.

Note: The swaddle should be snug but not overly tight. Your baby should be able to move his legs slightly, meaning that the swaddle should be loose around the hips. You should be able to place two or three fingers between the folds to make sure it's not too tight.

Baby Breathing Monitors: What You Should Know

These are devices with an alarm that goes off if your baby stops breathing. Pediatricians may recommend a breathing monitor for premature babies or babies who have breathing problems. Other than that, they're not essential when it comes to baby sleep safety.

You may opt to have a baby monitor even if your baby is normal. However, in my opinion, they can become an obsession and may lead to unnecessary middle of the night scares. Babies don't have regular breathing like adults when they sleep. They tend to have pauses in their breathing, which may set the monitor off. To say that these false alarms are stressful for parents is an understatement. They're downright terrifying. If you have a normal baby but are considering a breathing monitor nonetheless, it could be helpful to speak with your child's healthcare provider and consider their advice.

The Flat Spot on the Baby's Head

The heads of newborns are very soft. Nature created them that way so that they can pass out of the mother's womb during birth. As a result of sleeping on their backs, the back of their heads may become somewhat flat. The scientific term for this is positional plagiocephaly. This is often a cause for panic by parents, but it's normal and goes away by the time your baby is 12 months old.

You can avoid this by turning your baby's head to one side as he sleeps – but remember, always on his back. Give your baby plenty of time on his tummy when he's awake as well.

The Safe Sleep Seven

All of the above information can be summed up in 7 basic safe sleep rules, where your baby should:

1. Sleep on his back

2. Sleep in his crib

3. Sleep in a safe crib with the right bedding

4. Sleep in the proper sleepwear

5. Sleep in a well-ventilated room

6. Sleep in a bare crib with no pillows or blankets

7. Sleep without getting overheated

Takeaways

Safe sleep for your baby must always be your top priority. Creating a safe sleeping environment for your little one is pretty easy but goes a long way in preventing serious sleep accidents and SUDI.

Make sure your sleep safety techniques include: proper sleep position, proper sleep surface, proper sleepwear and bedding, avoiding overheating, and keeping your baby away from cigarette smoke. Sharing a room with your baby or sharing a bed if you need to can also be safe and comfortable for both of you with the right precautions in place.

Now that you're aware of these essential sleep procedures and the risks involved if you neglect them, there is no excuse for not putting these into place ASAP. Your baby will sleep more safely, and you'll sleep with more peace of mind.

CHAPTER 8

SLEEP PROMOTING FOODS
FOR BABY

H ave you ever heard of "brain foods"? They're called that because they contain nutrients that improve cognitive function and boost brainpower. Likewise, certain foods can promote sleep. This chapter will focus on "sleep foods" which contain powerful sleep-promoting properties. The earlier you train your baby to enjoy these foods, the better the chance they'll become a part of his diet for the rest of his life. But for our present purpose, they will help your baby sleep better.

Naturally, your newborn's sustenance is going to be formula or breastmilk for his first 4 or 5 months, but when he starts experimenting with food, you can start introducing these sleep foods to boost his sleep quality and calm his mood.

First, a word about baby formula and breastfeeding. Baby formula contains all the nutrients your baby needs to grow and develop but there's no way you can alter it or add anything to make your baby sleep better. However, if you're breastfeeding, there are ways to make your breast milk more sleep-friendly. Breast milk is not made from the food you eat but from your blood, which contains components of that food. Some of these components help your baby sleep better, while others may keep him awake.

How to Make Breast Milk More Sleep-Friendly for Your Baby

You may have noticed that after you have had a particularly rich meal, your baby falls into a "milk-drunk" sleep even as he's still nursing. The "richer" and more nutritious your breastmilk is, the better your baby will sleep. So, if you're breastfeeding, make sure you're giving your baby the best by looking after your nutrition.

- Drink plenty of liquids like fresh juices and herbal teas, and lots of water.

- Eat protein-rich foods like dairy products, lean meat, and eggs.

- Avoid spicy foods, which can cause your baby indigestion and keep him awake.

- Avoid foods that contain caffeine, including carbonated drinks, which can keep the baby alert.

■ Avoid sugar as much as you can as this can also cause sleeplessness in your baby.

Super Sleep-Boosting Foods for Your Baby

I t's fun introducing new foods to your baby and watching his reaction. He will either love something so much that he keeps his mouth open, eagerly waiting for the next spoonful, or zip his lips tightly if the taste isn't to his liking.

Thankfully, the list of sleep-fostering foods is varied and there should be several things on it that your baby will love.

Bananas

Babies love the sweet taste of bananas. They make a great pre-bedtime meal not only because they're filling, but they also contain a high concentration of magnesium, which is a muscle relaxant. Bananas also contain melatonin (the sleep hormone), and serotonin (the "feel-good" hormone), so they should relax your baby and put him in the perfect mood for sleep.

How to prepare: Peel a banana and puree it. You can add a tablespoon of fresh orange juice or milk for added taste and softness.

White Rice and Wheat

These are found in baby cereals like "Cerelac" and are highly nutritious for active and growing babies. A warm bowl before naptime or bedtime will make your baby's tummy feel happy and warm, and help him fall asleep faster – and stay asleep longer.

Spinach

Let's face it. This is one food that's difficult to get your baby to like. But spinach is packed with melatonin and can boost your baby's sleep. Your best bet is to mix it with other foods to make it more palatable for your baby.

How to prepare: Baby food that contains spinach along with other ingredients like chicken or veal is the simplest option. Boil and puree the spinach on its own to see if your baby will eat it that way, or add a piece of chicken breast (also sleep-promoting) to hide the flavor if your baby doesn't take to it.

Cherries

Babies love cherries! I never met one who didn't. This is great because they happen to be packed with melatonin.

How to prepare: Deseed some fresh cherries and puree. Tart cherries contain more melatonin so you can puree a banana with them to sweeten. Yum!

Chicken

Chicken is the best baby "comfort food" and also a baby favorite. Chicken is high in tryptophan, a sleep-promoting amino acid that induces drowsiness and relaxation. You can be sure that your baby will drift off to sleep after a nice chicken dinner.

How to prepare: Baby food chicken dinners are your best option as they come in a wide variety, like chicken and peas, chicken and potatoes or mixed vegetables, etc. Simply heat and serve for a delicious baby dinner.

Chickpeas

Chickpeas are high in nutrition as well as high in tryptophan. They can be served alone or pureed with other foods and most babies like the taste.

How to prepare: Boil the chickpeas until they are very soft and puree.

Dairy Products

The proverbial glass of milk before bedtime is based on fact. Dairy products promote drowsiness and sleep. You can start adding regular milk to your baby's diet at around 6 months, as well as organic yogurt. Pureed bananas with yogurt are an all-round baby favorite! As he nears the 12-month mark, introduce him to cheese.

Solid Food and Baby Sleep - What to Expect

The transition to eating solid food is a huge one for your baby and can affect his sleep as his body adapts to the new diet. Your baby may experience some digestive and some discomfort that could affect his sleep. His digestive system needs some time to adapt from a liquid diet to a varied one of solid foods. This will not last long and is a normal part of his development, so there's no cause for worry. Many babies adjust right from the start and their sleep is not affected at all. The transition might be improved by more filling and sleep-inducing food.

Introduce solid foods gradually in small quantities. For the first week or two, try experimenting with one or two new foods at a time. Don't overwhelm your baby with too many new tastes and flavors all at once. For the first couple of weeks, feed your baby solid foods during the day with his normal milk feed before bedtime. When your baby adapts, you can start feeding the sleep-promoting foods for his dinner.

Just as you have a fixed bedtime hour, have a fixed dinner hour. This should be about 1 to 1.5 hours before you put your baby to sleep. Your baby may experience some discomfort during the night and wake up more often, but this will quickly pass. "Tummy time" is an excellent way to prevent this.

What is Tummy Time?

Tummy time is a technique that has been proven by research to have several benefits, including helping babies sleep better. It's widely popular with young parents so if you're not familiar with it, it could be something to learn about and try with your little one.

For a while during each day, place your baby on his stomach while he is awake. There's no set time for this. You can leave him there as long as he's comfortable, but if he starts falling asleep, you must lay him on his back as we discussed earlier. During tummy time, a parent must always be present to supervise the baby.

Experts say that tummy time is a sort of tummy massage or gentle workout for a baby's abdominal area. It helps relieve gases, improve digestion and regulate that baby's bowel movements.

You can start tummy time with your baby as soon as he is born. It's safe. Naturally, a calm tummy leads to better sleep, and "tummy time" is a great technique to reinforce your child's sleep routine

Note: Never start tummy time immediately after meals.

Takeaways

Your baby's diet can play an important role in improving his sleep. Sleep-boosting foods are healthy, well-liked, and tolerated by most babies and are packed with sleep-friendly substances. What better way to help your baby ease into a new diet while helping him sleep better!

You can guide your baby into the transition more effectively with tummy time too. If this is a new concept to you, try it! The benefits are well worth it.

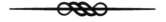

CHAPTER 9

TRAVEL AND BABY SLEEP

....

Having a new baby is not a prison sentence without parole. It doesn't mean staying within a 2-mile radius of your home until your child is old enough to start kindergarten.

Smart parenting means striking a good balance between your baby's routines and your regular activities and family needs - and that includes trips.

Now, I don't mean driving out for a quick dinner, a hasty trip to the grocery store, or a walk in the local park with baby in his stroller. I mean the wide-open spaces and the uncharted seas...I'm talking about travel. I mean travel in every sense of the word, as in booking a hotel, driving cross-country, going on a cruise, or boarding an airplane for a vacation in Italy!

Some parents may be horrified by this idea. Traveling with a baby in tow? That would be a nightmare! Where would he sleep? What if he gets sick? How would you manage a consistent feeding and sleeping routine? What if he doesn't stop crying and fussing? These are the kinds of thoughts that typically race through parents' minds when you suggest travel.

The truth is, most babies are perfect angels when it comes to travel. They take it in their stride and adapt very quickly indeed, with a little help from you. Traveling with your baby is a perfectly viable option and relatively hassle-free. It can be just the sanity-saving timeout you need.

Understandably, your biggest fear is that your baby's sleep routine will be disrupted and that you'll have to start all over again when you get home - this isn't true.

With a few smart preparations and tweaks, you create a home away from home for your baby. This chapter will walk you through the steps of how you and your baby can enjoy traveling together. So, read on and start planning that holiday!

Where Will Your Baby Sleep?

This is the first question that every parent asks. They start to panic because they fear that their baby will cry and fuss if his sleeping environment changes. Naturally, nothing can replace your baby's crib and home sleeping environment, so a little flexibility is required here. With a little extra cuddling and settling, your baby will adapt to a new sleeping space in a day or two.

Whether you are staying in someone's house or in a hotel, you'll find that one of the following alternatives will work very well.

1. Portable Travel Crib

This is such a great option. A travel crib is easy to set up and disassemble. It will fit perfectly in a corner of your room to give your baby his own little sleeping niche. If you think this is a good option, there are dozens of safe and relatively inexpensive brands on the market.

Check out some of the best choices here:

▶ http://bit.ly/bestravelcribs

Unfortunately, there's a catch. Travel cribs can be somewhat heavy and cumbersome. If you're traveling in your truck, that shouldn't be an issue. But these types of cribs may not be suitable for air travel. You'll have to lug them through airports plus play extra for transport. However, if your trip is an extended one, it may be worth the trouble and cost.

2. Hotel Crib

Many hotels are baby-friendly and happy to accommodate your baby by providing a crib. These include many of the major hotel chains as well as mid-scale hotels. You can easily arrange this when making the booking to ensure that your baby's crib is ready and waiting in your room. One thing to remember is that hotel cribs tend to be on the smaller side, so do ask for details if you're traveling with a toddler. Also, make sure the room is big enough for the crib so that you're not climbing over things to move around.

When some hotels say that they provide a crib, that may mean a travel crib or a compact crib. Just be clear on the details so that you know what to expect. Always inspect the hotel crib and make sure the mattress fits snugly and is firm, and that the sheet is clean. Wipe down the crib thoroughly with disinfectant wipes and welcome the baby to his new sleeping space!

3. Sleeping Pod

This sounds like something out of a science fiction movie but it's a sort of glorified sleeping sack. It's sometimes called a "baby nest" or cocoon. The sleeping pod resembles a little nest or tent with a flat, thin sleeping surface surrounded by a soft, fluffy enclosure. I know a lot of people who use them as kitty-beds as well!

Baby pods are a big trend these days and babies love them. For travel, they're much lighter and compact than portable cribs. However, you will have to put it on the floor of your room and place your baby in it which may not be a very safe option. I must also warn you that there is some controversy over the overall safety of baby pods. Some experts suggest that they may be a suffocation hazard while others claim that they are safe. There is no research to back up either side as of yet.

I would suggest, however, that you could bring a baby pod on your trips and use it for naps, where the baby can sleep in your bed while you are supervising. It could also be used for tummy time or awake time, also under your supervision.

4. Bed-Sharing

Of course, just sharing your bed with your baby is the simplest option but it really should be your last choice. If you do decide to share your bed with the baby, please make sure that you follow the experts' advice by placing him in a bassinet with a firm, flat surface that acts as a buffer between you and your baby. This is especially important for newborns up to 6 months. Also, make sure (beforehand if possible) that the bed is big enough for parents and baby to sleep comfortably.

Baby's Sleep Routine - Pick Up Where You Left Off

Your main concern when traveling with your baby is the disruption of his sleep routine which you've both worked so hard to keep consistent.

Your baby needs one or two days to adapt to his new environment, but his routine need not be disrupted if you pick up where you left off. This means doing all the familiar things your baby is used to. Below, you will find some of them.

Bedtimes, Nap Times, and Feeding Times

Just bring your normal home schedule along with you. Stick to your baby's regular sleep hours and nap times and follow the same feeding schedule you had at home. This may take a little effort and sometimes might not be possible, so be flexible when you need to and don't sweat. Just try to be consistent in a loose kind of way, if that makes sense!

Don't worry if you can't follow the schedule like clockwork. As soon as you get home, your baby will immediately readjust to his normal schedule without fuss and fall back into his regular sleep habits.

Sleepsack

Bring along your baby's beloved sleep sack and he'll feel right at home. He'll have no trouble falling asleep.

A good idea is to pack two sleep sacks; a light one and a heavier one. Remember, you may not be able to control the room temperature as you do at home, and it's much easier to switch sleep sacks than ask the hotel or your host to adjust the temperature.

Resume Tummy Time!

If tummy time is a familiar routine for your baby, nothing can be simpler than resuming it. There should be a safe place in your room where you can do this.

Using a couch is okay if you are sitting next to your baby. Otherwise, place him in his crib or in a baby pod for some nice (and familiar) tummy time.

Sleep Boosting Foods

Pack a few jars of your baby's favorite sleep-boosting foods. You may not be able to find them easily or just not have the time to shop while on holiday. Having them handy will save you a lot of headaches and will mean that your baby can continue to eat the same foods he did at home.

Additionally, the sleep-promoting properties of these foods will be more useful than ever to help your baby sleep better in his new surroundings.

White Noise Machine

If your baby's used to being soothed to sleep by some kind of white noise, buy a white noise machine. It can be placed under his crib or near his sleeping space to create his familiar ambiance.

The same applies to lullabies or storybooks. Bring along a recording of your little one's favorite lullabies to play on your phone or pack a couple of storybooks.

Inflatable Baby Bathtub

If a warm bath is a regular part of your baby's bedtime routine, you need to get an inflatable bathtub. It's much safer and more hygienic than bathing him in the hotel sink or bathtub. Inflatable baby tubs are inexpensive, durable, and easy to pack. They're a great addition to any baby travel gear.

Favorite Comfort Toy

Bring along your baby's favorite stuffed toy to keep him company. If snuggling with his furry pal is part of his routine, he can easily do that. The comfort of having his favorite toy with him will soothe him right to sleep.

Baby Sleep Items to Consider When Traveling

In addition to bringing items that help you carry on with your home sleep routine, you may also want to bring along the following:

Bassinet

A bassinet is great for air travel as it means you don't have to carry your baby throughout the flight. He will also feel more comfortable sleeping in a bassinet.

Stroller

A stroller is a must if you're going to be doing a lot of walking or sightseeing, and it doubles as a crib. You can easily feed and settle your baby in his stroller, and he can sleep while you stroll.

Blanket

A blanket can be handy for covering your baby in his stroller or covering the stroller itself to filter out light as he sleeps.

Portable shade

This could come in handy to place over a window and provide sufficient darkness for your baby to sleep.

Baby's Crib Sheet from Home

A baby's sense of smell is very developed. He'll be able to detect the familiar smell of home on the sheet, which can have a soothing effect. The familiar scent of his sleeping environment can be found in his sleep sack as well.

Portable Monitor

If you're staying with family or trusted friends, a portable baby monitor is good for supervising your baby when you're not in the room. I do not recommend ever leaving your baby alone in a hotel room, so a portable baby monitor isn't necessary for hotel stays.

Avoid Starting Bad Sleep Habits

Flexibility is essential when you're traveling, but you need to draw the line at allowing your baby to form new (bad) sleep habits. It will take you ages to get him back on track because habits are much harder to break than a flexible compromise here and there.

For example, if your baby is trained to fall asleep in his crib, never go back to rocking and cuddling him in your arms until he falls asleep. If he's fussing and crying, settle and cuddle him repeatedly but always put him back in his crib to sleep.

If your baby is partially night weaned, don't nurse him outside of his usual feeding times in order to soothe him to sleep. No matter how frustrating this may be, never be tempted to take the easy way out. Think how much tougher it will be once you return home and have to start sleep training all over again.

Baby Sleep and Jet Lag

If you're traveling by air, here are the basic facts about jet lag and baby–lag; yes, babies get jet lag too! Depending on how long the trip is, babies need 2-3 days to get over jet lag, after which they'll return to their normal sleep patterns. During this time, your baby will be fussier than usual and have difficulty falling asleep and staying asleep. He will also want to be close to you and fuss if you're not near. Unfortunately, jet lag can't be prevented. Your only option is to tough it out. But you can help your baby quickly get back on track and make these few days easier by starting your child's sleep routine as soon as you arrive.

Try to be as consistent as possible so that your baby falls back into his normal sleep patterns ASAP. Jet lag is not dangerous for babies, just a bit of an inconvenience for you.

Takeaways

Hopefully, this chapter has demonstrated that it's not that hard to pack up your baby's sleep routine and take it with you wherever you go. Traveling with a baby is well worth it and the inconvenience is minor if you're well-prepared and willing to be a bit flexible.

So, start planning that vacation and give your baby some early travel experience. This first time is the hardest. But when travel becomes a normal part of your baby's life, he'll soon become a pro at adapting to any sleeping situations.

CHAPTER 10

SOLVING BABY SLEEP PROBLEMS

New parents hear a lot of stories from other parents that can cause confusion and worry. They start to wonder if their baby's sleep patterns are normal. There are stories about "angel babies" who hardly ever cry, fall straight to sleep after nursing, and never give Mommy and Daddy a hard time. Then there are the horror stories about babies who cry nonstop, wake up every hour throughout the night and take ages to fall asleep. So, what's normal and what's not? Could your baby have serious sleep problems?

First of all, there's no such thing as a serious sleep problem, at least not one that is life-threatening for a baby. An underlying medical issue could disrupt a baby's sleep but that's another matter altogether. I think most babies fall somewhere in between those two extremes. Even with a sleep routine in place, babies have their good days and their bad ones. They'll be perfect angels some days and terrible tormentors on others.

So, what's the point of a sleep routine? It will breed consistency! It will help your baby ease out of any sleep problems and ease into a regular sleep pattern.

This chapter will discuss the most common baby sleep problems and offer solutions.

Baby and Toddler Sleep Concerns

Despite having a good sleep routine in place, your baby may continue to have some sleep issues. Below, I've listed the most common ones and how to deal with them.

Baby Will not Follow a Napping Schedule or Fall Asleep for Naps

If your baby sleeps normally during the night but struggles to settle down for a nap, this is perfectly normal. Believe it or not, this is an indication that your sleep routine has been pretty successful! It means your baby has learned to associate nighttime with sleep and as a result, finds it hard to sleep during the day. The solution lies in some additional nap training.

Here's how:

- Be extra alert to tiredness signs and immediately start the nap routine, even if your baby resists.

- Keep your baby active so that he expends more energy and is ready to get some rest at naptime.

- Make sure your baby's sleeping space is as dark as possible during the day. Heavy blackout curtains will do the trick.

- Use familiar bedtime activities for naptime, like white noise, lullabies, and storytelling. A warm bath can also help relax the baby when he's being overly hyperactive and irritable.

- Feed your baby a filling lunch or snack containing one of the sleep-promoting foods discussed earlier.

- Take a bit longer to settle and soothe your baby until he starts falling asleep.

Settling your baby for naps can sometimes take longer than it does for night sleep if he's resisting naptime. As frustrating as this can be, it's essential for your baby to get enough rest during the day, especially as he becomes more active. Never skip nap times or have an irregular schedule. Be patient! The above tips will gradually ease your child into napping consistently and without fuss.

Baby Resists Sleeping on His Back

This is when your baby fusses, cries, and kicks when you lay him on his back to sleep. Conversely, he quiets when placed on his tummy. Babies feel safer when sleeping on their stomachs, but as we've learned, this is a big no-no. Never give in to your baby on this one.

What to do:

- Swaddling a baby will gradually help him fall asleep on his back. A sleeping sack could work as well. However, swaddling may be a better option for this problem because it constricts a baby's movements better while calming and soothing him. Remember to gradually phase out swaddling so that it doesn't become a habit.

- A pacifier could distract your baby and soothe him to sleep.

- Consult your pediatrician. Although this is a common problem among many babies, there could be underlying issues causing real discomfort to the baby.

Sleep Regression

Your sleep routine is going great. Your baby is falling asleep on time, waking up less at night and going back to sleep with minimum fuss. You give yourself a big pat on the back, thinking the worst is over… then suddenly, at around 4 months, the baby decides he hates sleeping and that he's going to avoid it as much as he can!

This is another common problem called sleep regression. It happens at around 4 months, 6 months, and 10 months, and it's totally normal. What causes it? Your baby's becoming more active and more alert to all the awesome things around him.

He's flexing his body and discovering new ways to move it. He's starting to recognize familiar toys and surroundings. His senses are bursting with new sounds, tastes, and smells. Who wants to waste time sleeping when there's so much cool stuff to be explored? Yes, babies are smart enough to make the deduction that less sleep means more fun, but of course they're not aware that sleep is vital to their health and development.

What to do:

▦ Stick to your bedtime routine. Be patient but firm and let your baby know you mean business. Bedtimes and nap times are not going to go away. When your baby objects, settle him as many times as needed, but always place him in his crib and leave the room.

▦ Don't skip naps. The more active your baby gets, the more (not less) naptime becomes important. Overtiredness plus sleep regression will make it even harder to get your baby to sleep at night.

▦ Add more sleep-boosting foods to your child's diet in various combinations for more potency. Bananas pureed with warm milk or baby cereal with a mashed banana should help your baby wind down.

Relax! Sleep regression is temporary and won't wreck your sleep training. Your baby will fall right back into his sleep routine in a week or so.

Baby Will not Fall Asleep on His Own

The whole point of sleep training is to get your baby to self-settle and drift off on his own. But when you start the bedtime routine everything is fine until you settle him in his crib and start to leave the room. He starts crying and will not fall asleep unless you are sitting or standing nearby.

What to do:

- Tweak your bedtime routine with longer cuddling and comfort time lullabies and baby massage until your baby gets drowsy before placing him in his crib. Be careful not to let him fall asleep in your arms.

- Try nursing your baby with breastmilk or a bottle 30 minutes before bed.

- Allow your baby to self-settle and fall asleep with a pacifier.

- Swaddling can be very effective in this situation.

As long as your baby learns to fall asleep on his own at bedtime, it's okay to pick him up for a cuddle if he wakes up during the night. This is the best way to ease out of this problem. Next, you can just walk into the room and soothe him only with your voice.

Baby Falls Asleep Only When Swaddled

Swaddling is a good way to soothe a baby to sleep, but when it becomes the only way you can get him to drift off, it becomes a bad sleep habit.

What to do:

- Partial night swaddling: Swaddle the baby for bed and let him drift off to sleep. When you're sure, he's sleeping soundly, unwrap the swaddling. When he wakes up for his next feeding, try settling him without a swaddle with a lot of cuddles and soothing whispers. As your baby sleeps for longer periods during the night without being swaddled, it will cease being a problem.

- Try swaddling your baby with one arm out of the swaddle for a night or two. Next, leave both arms out for another night or two. When he becomes accustomed to this, continue with partial swaddling, where you unwrap the legs as he sleeps.

- Use a swaddle strap: This is a small swaddle that only wraps around your baby's arms and chest. It will give him the same comfort and you can gradually wean him by unwrapping it as he sleeps.

Colic

We briefly discussed colic earlier, but more details are needed here since this is a problem that can be extremely disruptive to a baby's sleep.

About 25% of newborns suffer from colic, which starts at birth. The symptoms typically reach their peak at 4-6 weeks and last up to 3-4 months. The intensity and frequency of the attacks gradually decline and disappear completely by the time the baby is 9 months old.

The causes of colic are unknown but the most common theory is gas and digestive problems caused by swallowing too much air while nursing. It's not life-threatening or dangerous for the baby but it can cause extreme discomfort.

Recognize Colic Symptoms?

If your child displays the following symptoms, he may be experiencing colic. You must take him to his pediatrician to confirm this:

- Clenched fists

- Passing gas

- Crying

- Jerking arms and legs towards the stomach.

- Red, flushed face

- Bloated stomach

The symptoms will be heightened in the evening and during the night, disrupting the baby's sleep.

Is There a Cure for Colic?

There is no safe medication to treat colic. Should your pediatrician prescribe one, be sure to ask the right questions and perhaps seek a second opinion before giving it to your baby. Your pediatrician may, however, prescribe a natural remedy like the famous Gripe Water, which has been safely used to calm colic in generations of babies. It's not a miracle cure but is known to ease some colic symptoms.

You can also try the following:

- Swaddling your baby with his legs slightly flexed.

- Rocking your baby in your arms to soft music (sound and motion have been known to ease colic).

- Changing the baby's formula.

■ Using a pacifier.

How Does Colic Affect Your Baby's Sleep Routine?

C olic may seriously impact your baby's ability to sleep, much less have a consistent sleep routine.

So where does that leave you? My best advice is to start a sleep routine but be prepared to be flexible - very flexible, as in skipping it altogether on days when your baby is in too much discomfort. This is probably the most convenient option for you and your baby.

It's nearly impossible to settle a colicky baby in his crib. The more you try, the more distressed he will become. Rocking him to sleep in your arms will be less stressful for you both. On other days when your baby is feeling better, a normal sleep routine can go off without a hitch.

Remember, your little one is in real distress here. If he needs to be rocked, cuddled, and given extra loving care, his well-being must always come first. There's plenty of time to train your baby more consistently. What matters most now is that Mommy and Daddy are always there to make it better.

Teething and Nighttime Troubles

A re those first teeth sprouting and your baby can't sleep well for the pain? Teething is an unavoidable part of your baby's development. It can happen at any time, day or night (but at least during the day, you expect to be awake).

To avoid states of nighttime restlessness, both for the newborn and for you, it is good to know how teething works and how to remedy it effectively.

Most babies begin teething somewhere between 4 and 7 months of age, though it can happen earlier or later. Some of the most common symptoms of teething include:

- Irritability or crankiness

- Excessive drooling

- Chewing on solid objects

- Sore or tender gums (next to the coming tooth)

- One cheek is flushed

- They are rubbing their ear or cheek

- They continually bring their hands to their mouth

There is no direct relationship between teething and the following symptoms: high fever, diarrhea, or anything else not mentioned on the above list. If your baby exhibits these other symptoms, you should speak with your child's pediatrician.

So, what can you do to calm your little one down and bring him back to the dream world at night so both of you can enjoy some rest?

Best 6 Ways to Soothe Teething

- **Rub your Baby's gums:** rub your baby's gums softly using a clean finger; the pressure can ease discomfort.

- **Keep it cool:** use a teething ring, a spoon, or a cold washcloth to soothe your baby's gums. The temperature should be cool but not freezing, or you will get the opposite effect.

- **Offer a teething ring:** these are more effective if made of firmer rubber. If you don't have one, you can use his feeding bottle filled with water.

- **Try hard foods:** if your baby is eating solid foods, you may give him something edible for gnawing (peeled and chilled carrot, or cucumber). Always keep an eye out for little parts, as they can pose a choking hazard.

- **Dry the drool:** keep a clean cloth handy in order to dry your baby's chin. Teething can cause excessive drooling.

- **Try an over-the-counter remedy:** if your baby is very cranky, you can help him with acetaminophen or ibuprofen, but be sure to avoid teething medications containing benzocaine. Remember to ask to your baby's pediatrician if you think medication is needed.

Teething, like many other periods in your baby's life is a temporary situation. No matter how tempting it might be to suspend your baby's regular bedtime routine, don't do it!

Phasing Out Negative Sleep Associations

B aby sleep training can be tricky, especially for first-time parents. In the process of night weaning and teaching your baby to self-settle, there's a possibility that he might make some negative sleep associations. Let's find out what these are and how to phase them out.

Positive vs. Negative Sleep Associations

S leep associations are any action related to sleep. Adults, as well as babies, have sleep associations. For example, praying before bedtime, reading, or having a glass of milk. Babies learn to make these associations very early on. For them it's like learning a very basic math equation: Darkness = Sleep, or Mommy nursing me = Sleep, or Daddy rocking me = Sleep.

A negative sleep association is when the baby relies on something other than himself to go to sleep - namely, you! A positive sleep association is where the baby relies on himself to fall asleep.

Some examples of negative sleep associations are:

- Nursing a baby to sleep.

- Rocking a baby to sleep.

- Picking up and nursing/cradling the baby each time he wakes up crying.

- Pushing the baby in a stroller until he falls asleep.

- Allowing the baby to sleep in the parents' bed.

- Feeding a baby each time he wakes up.

Now here are some examples of positive sleep associations:

- Sucking the thumb or the fingers.

- Sucking a pacifier.

- Humming or singing to himself.

- Moving back and forth

- Banging against the mattress with his legs.

- Body rocking and head-rolling.

- Blackout curtains.

White noise or nature sounds.

A good sleep routine helps your baby make positive associations. This is why the emphasis should be on ramping up to the point where you place the baby in his crib before he is asleep. The faster you can phase out rocking or nursing him to sleep, the less likely he will associate these activities with sleep.

Pacifiers and Sleep Associations

There's some controversy around whether "dummies" or pacifiers can create negative sleep associations. Many babies find sucking on a dummy very soothing and oftentimes, it's the easiest way to get a baby to fall asleep on his own. If this is the case with your baby, go ahead and use a dummy, but bear in mind the following:

Try to limit dummy use to nighttime sleep but not for naps.

Use a dummy only for sleep. Don't let your baby keep it in his mouth during his waking hours.

Phase-out the use of a dummy by decreasing its use when the baby wakes up during the night. Try to settle him without it.

Always remove the dummy from your baby's mouth after he falls asleep.

129

Controlled Comforting Strategy

Controlled comforting is the key to encouraging independent sleep in your baby. It's the most effective way to ease your baby out of a negative parent-sleep association and avoid unhealthy separation anxiety.

Controlled comforting, as we discussed earlier, is where you place your baby in his crib, soothe him until he's quiet, and then leave the room. Here is a more detailed description of the steps to take:

- It all starts with a positive bedtime routine that puts your baby in the perfect mood for sleep.

- When you decide to begin controlled comfort, take a little bit longer with the bedtime routine to fully relax your baby.

- When your baby becomes drowsy, place him in the crib and comfort him by making soothing noises and patting him for one minute.

- Say goodnight and leave the room while the baby is still awake.

- Listen to your baby's response. If he starts fussing but not crying hard, don't go back into the room; give him time to settle.

- If your baby starts to cry, wait for two minutes then go back into the room and repeat the controlled comforting. Each time your baby starts crying, increase the intervals before you go into the room (3, 4, 5 minutes, with 6 being the maximum).

▨ Each time you enter the room, comfort and pat your baby in the same way for 2-3 minutes or until he is quiet.

▨ Try not to pick up your baby and cuddle him but if you are both becoming too distressed, it's okay to do so.

▨ When your baby is crying, wait for the specified interval before going in, but try talking to him from outside the room to see if he quiets down.

▨ Stick to it and your baby will slowly learn to fall asleep on his own.

When to Stop Controlled Comforting

There are times when controlled comforting should be stopped temporarily for the sake of you and your baby's wellbeing. You can easily pick up where you left off in a day or two. Controlled comforting should be stopped when:

▨ Your baby is ill with a cough or cold.

▨ On particularly stressful days when you are too exhausted and impatient.

- When you are traveling and have to share a bed with your baby.

- When your baby is teething.

- If your baby has colic.

Takeaways

No sleep routine goes off without a hitch. It can come with its own set of problems specific to your baby's temperament. Thankfully, most sleep problems are common to babies and are easily tackled.

For new parents, baby sleep training is an art that needs to be mastered through trial and error, as well as some creativity. It can be a balancing act between training your baby to sleep independently without creating negative associations. It can be overwhelming when you've control-comforted your baby for the tenth time and he still won't stop crying.

Always remember that it's a labor of love. Be patient and stick to it. The amazing results you'll begin to see and expect to see will be all the motivation you need to keep going!

CONCLUSION

Putting it all Together

Congratulations! You are officially a very well-informed parent on the dynamics of baby sleep! If this book has fulfilled its purpose, you are now able to see the bigger picture of how all of these tips and methods come together to create a powerful set of sleep habits. By easing your baby into good sleep habits, you are setting him up for a lifetime of good health.

You now understand the importance of having a great sleep routine for your baby, and how it will instill healthy lifelong sleep habits. You are well-informed about baby sleep risks and how to create the safest possible sleeping environment for your little one. You are well-equipped to travel with your baby with minimum disruption to his sleep routine and are ready to tackle any sleep problems he may have. To top it all, you have a list of yummy sleep-boosting foods that will help your baby adapt even better.

Now, it's time to take action! Start creating a sleep routine and a safe environment for your baby today. Everything else will come together and fall into place as you progress. Experiment a bit with the various methods suggested here until you find what works best for your baby. Make little changes as your baby grows. And most importantly of all, stay consistent!

Good health starts with good sleep. By creating a consistent sleep routine, you are preparing your baby for a lifetime of healthy sleep habits. What's more, he's likely to instill the same habits in his children one day. Imagine that - your legacy will extend to your grandchildren as well! Creating the perfect sleep routine goes beyond good parenting. It's a priceless labor of love.

Finally, this book has been a labor of love on my part as well. My goal was to provide a comprehensive but simple guide that would cover everything parents need to train their baby for quality sleep. I hope I've succeeded! I understand how awesome but overwhelming caring for a new baby can be and how a baby's sleep can be the biggest challenge parents face.

My greatest wish is that all parents, and even parents-to-be, will read this book and realize the importance of baby sleep training. More importantly, I want you to realize how easy it is to instill these habits in your baby early on, with nothing but some patience and flexibility.

If you enjoyed the book, please recommend it to others and express your thoughts and feedback by writing a short review on the site where you purchased it.

I love hearing from my readers and take every comment and feedback seriously. I look forward to engaging with you again…

Thank You!

Lisa Marshall

SCAN ME TO LEAVE A REVIEW

HAPPY PARENTING AND SWEET

DREAMS FOR YOUR BABY!

ALSO BY

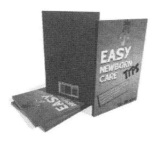

Easy Newborn Care Tips - Proven Parenting Tips For Your Newborn's Development, Sleep Solution And Complete Feeding Guide

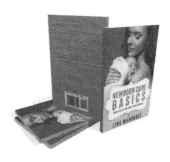

Newborn Care Basics: Baby Care Tips For New Moms

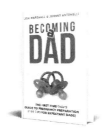

<u>Becoming a Dad: The First-Time Dad's Guide to Pregnancy Preparation (101 Tips For Expectant Dads)</u>

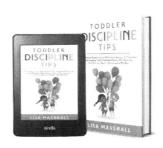

<u>Toddler Discipline Tips: The Complete Parenting Guide With Proven Strategies To Understand And Managing Toddler's Behavior, Dealing With Tantrums, And Reach An Effective Communication With Kids</u>

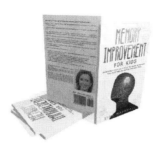

Memory Improvement For Kids: The Greatest Collection Of Proven Techniques For Expanding Your Child's Mind And Boosting Their Brain Power (Montessori Parenting Book 1)

BONUS

Want more?

Get a FREE Audiobook on my series with Audible.

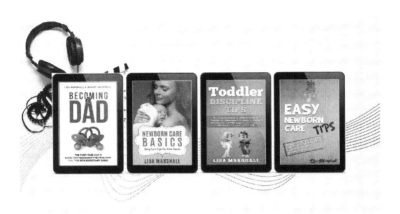

Scan this code with your phone!

YOUR FREE GIFT

Thank you for purchasing this book. Click on this link to download this free tool.

http://bit.ly/BabySelfSooth

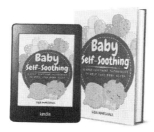

This tool is a useful resource to help your baby being able to self-soothe themselves to sleep. We've compiled some tips to help make the process as quick as possible!

Scan this code with your phone!

Bibliography

(n.d.). Retrieved from Babyology.com: https://babyology.com.au/baby/sleeping/9-ways-to-create-the-perfect-sleep-environment-for-your-baby

(n.d.). Retrieved from Mom365.com: https://www.mom365.com/baby/baby-gear/how-to-choose-the-right-baby-bedding

(n.d.). Retrieved from Secondlife.com: https://www.mother.ly/child/8-tips-for-setting-up-a-sleep-inducing-nursery/1-limit-light-sources

10 Things to Hate About Sleep Loss. (n.d.). Retrieved from WebMD: https://www.webmd.com/sleep-disorders/features/10-results-sleep-loss

50 Fascinating Facts About Sleep. (n.d.). Retrieved from Nature's Sleep: https://www.naturessleep.com/blog/50-fascinating-facts-about-sleep

9 Funny quotes about parenting and sleep. (n.d.). Retrieved from https://www.nanit.com/blog/9-funny-quotes-parenting-sleep/

Are Heaters Safe for Babies? (n.d.). Retrieved from https://www.mrright.in/ideas/appliances/room-heater/room-heaters-safe-babies-find/

Baby Sleep 2-12 Months. (n.d.). Retrieved from Raisingchildren.net: https://raisingchildren.net.au/babies/sleep/understanding-sleep/sleep-2-12-months

Baby Sleep Training: Night Weaning. (n.d.). Retrieved from Baby Center: https://www.babycenter.com/baby/sleep/baby-sleep-training-night-weaning

Baby Tummy Time. (n.d.). Retrieved from Vert Well Family: https://www.verywellfamily.com/importance-of-tummy-time-for-my-baby

Baby Sleep. (n.d.). Retrieved from https://kidslymom.com/newborn-sleep-schedule/

Five Stages of Sleep. (n.d.). Retrieved from https://www.healthy-eating-and-living-tips.com/five-stages-of-sleep.html

Newborn sleep routines. (n.d.). Retrieved from Familydoctor.org: https://familydoctor.org/newborn-sleep-routines/

Night weaning. (n.d.). Retrieved from Healthline: https://www.healthline.com/health/baby/night-weaning

Night Weaning. (n.d.). Retrieved from S, art Parent Advice: https://smartparentadvice.com/night-weaning/

What is Sleep Hygiene? (n.d.). Retrieved from Sleep Foundation: https://www.sleepfoundation.org/articles/sleep-hygiene

What to Expect for Newborn Sleep. (n.d.). Retrieved from https://familysleepinstitute.com/2020/08/17/what-to-expect-for-newborn-sleep/

Tired Signs in Babies. (n.d.). Retrieved from Raidongchildren.net: https://raisingchildren.net.au/babies/sleep/understanding-sleep/tired

Printed in Great Britain
by Amazon

64396458R00087